To: Chinedu

Medical Residency

Guide For The

International Graduate

What you need to know before you apply

Volume 1

OLAREWAJU OLADIPO, MD, MBA
YETUNDE KARE-OPANEYE MBBS

FOREWORD

I thank you for getting a copy of the Medical Residency Guide for the International Graduate - Volume 1.

I believe by the time you read the majority of the pages of this book, you would have obtained more in value than the amount of money you have spent in making its purchase. While this book was written with the international medical graduate in mind, a significant portion of it will apply to all those in the process of applying for residency training. Writing with a focus on the international medical graduate allows the authors to address many of the issues peculiar to this group.

The motivation to write this book arose out of the observation that year after year, new arrivals to the United States, and applicants interested in applying to medical residency training programs in the United States make the same mistakes. This observation is well supported by the seminars that we have coordinated over the years, and the many one-on-one sessions with several international graduates.

While this book does not guarantee you a better score on your United States Medical Licensing Examinations (USMLE), it offers you a better understanding of how to fulfill your ultimate goal irrespective of your test performance.

This book also serves as a starting point to make logical discussions with others, and identify areas that you need to work on in fulfilling that goal of a successful Match.

INTRODUCTION

One unique aspect of this publication is that many sections are supported by short stories, all of which are works of fiction. This approach was used to further reinforce the wisdom that this book promise to share. While you as a reader, like many others, may want to get straight to the points being offered, without the wisdom shared through these stories, many end up missing the real lessons that is intended to be learned. I believe you as a reader will have many more real life stories specific to several aspects of this phase of your career that you can share with others.

With combined years of experience of the authors in their roles as mentors and advisors to many international medical graduates, many stories have been heard of applicants with unique experiences in their quests to pass the necessary examinations, and to obtain training position. Many of these stories are ones of positive experiences, some which are hard to believe, and fit more in the realm of fiction, while others are unpleasant experiences that you would never wish on a colleague.

In the roles played in the numerous encounters with international medical graduates, most of whom are of the West African descent, as a listener and a sounding board, we have had a share of the emotions surrounding the whole process – from passing the necessary examination to successfully entering a residency training program. Some of the emotions that accompany the preparation for the examinations relate to the fear and insecurities. Personally, these encounters have been a wholesome learning experience in our role, one that has made us more committed in the desire to continue to play a positive role on the few international graduates that come our way.

The one thing that is constant in the process of securing training positions is that of changes - both in the design of the various licensing examinations, and the requirements for applying to a residency program. Despite all the changes that have been witnessed over the years, the essence of the exercise has remained the same that is to attain a competitive score in the examinations, and to successfully obtain a position for residency training. By focusing on these ultimate goals, it is much easier to navigate the various changes, and seek out how best to utilize them to your advantage.

While there is a lot to talk about, every attempt has been made to make the writing of this book as concise as possible. I sincerely wish you the best in your effort to secure a residency training position.

ACKNOWLEDGEMENT

This book is dedicated to all international medical graduates.

CONTENT

COMING TO AMERICA - HOW DO I GET THERE?

Every international medical graduate that end up in the United States often starts with this question. This question is considered a good starting point for this book, and one that is well illustrated in this short story.

It's five o'clock on a Monday morning in the middle of winter. I had just finished shoveling the snow in my driveway and was out of breath as I got hold of my mobile phone that has been securely placed on the front seat of my Toyota Camry. It was the longest I had been without the gadget all day, and I could not wait to get hold of it once I cleared the long stretch of snow. My first instinct was to check for any emails that had come in as I was expecting a notification on an order of a pair of glasses I had ordered. I did get an email of course, but not quite the one I was expecting. It was from Nigeria, written by a young female physician about to complete her year of compulsory National Service.

I read the email with a subdued interest, and browse for other emails that may have preceded hers, but there was none. I then returned to read the content of her email.

'I would like to come to the US for postgraduate training. I have no relatives in America, but it's my heart's desire to travel out of this country. I will be done with my current posting in three months and I have saved enough money to buy the ticket to travel. Kindly advise me. Yours truly, Adeshua.'

I was not totally surprised to get the email. I get about ten of such emails every month since I gave a seminar at a local university several months ago on the opportunities to train in the United States and why it is not impossible despite all the barriers and seemingly impossible limitations. In as much I wish I could ignore some of the emails that I receive, I make an effort to respond to every email, even if it is a one-line response.

My first email response was the beginning of a series of emails that detail Adeshua's journey from the moment she first contacted me until she finally arrived in the United States. I did not actually respond to her first email until about a week later. I had totally forgotten and was responding to another inquiry when her name flashed back into my memory. I decided to pen down a brief response before I forget again, and hoped that I would not hear again from her, as it is the case with many with a half-hearted desire to travel to the United States.

'Dear Adeshua, thank you for your email. There is more to coming to America than having your ticket fare. Do you have a travel visa and a right one at

that? How do you plan to survive before you start your postgraduate training? How much do you know about medical training in America? Is your medical school accredited for postgraduate training in the US? Do you have any idea of challenges you may encounter in your quest to get residency training in the US and how to deal with them? Have you given some of these questions any thought?"

This email from Adeshua is not that uncommon in my experience. The majority of emails that come my way take the same shape or form, and all have the common theme of the desire to come to America. In fact if all the medical graduates who had sent me emails in the past had been able to come over to the United States, they would fit the medical doctors need of a small town. Sometimes I wonder why some people end up achieving that dream of coming to the United States, and some people don't. What I discovered that separates those who did, and those who did not are their sheer determination and persistence. Adeshua was one of the few that were very determined and persistent in her effort to fulfill her goal, as you would find out in the rest of this story.

Contrary to my expectation, I got a response to my email in less than an hour after I sent it. I read about the beginning of my lunch break, and while I was waiting for my drink of tea to cool down, so I had a few minutes to read her rather lengthy email. Below is an excerpt of the email

'Dear Sir, thank you for your email. I never expected a reply.........since my last email to you; I had gone to research the first steps I needed to take before even considering traveling. It's obvious that three months is a very short time to meet the requirements. I would like to keep in touch as I make further plans in this direction. Yours truly, Adeshua'

I quickly realized that her email was not one of those emails that I could respond to in a hurry, especially with the way my schedule was for the rest of the day. Instead, I forwarded her email to my assistant to prioritize for discussion and consideration for guidance. Later that week, I sent a compilation of various websites that would offer valuable information more than I could ever cover in one email. The following is a list of the sites sent in that communication:

- http://www.usmle.org
- http://www.ecfmg.org
- http://www.faimer.org/resources/imed.html
- https://en.wikipedia.org/wiki/International_medical_graduate

The list was limited to a few considering the wealth of information that is available on the listed websites and to avoid the risk of her being lured into frivolous websites that offer promises of getting over to the United States for a fee.

TIPS/LESSONS

The best move made by Adeshua is the fact that she decided to embark on the process relatively early, approximately one to two years following graduation from medical school. It is common knowledge among international medical graduates that the longer it is since you graduated out of medical school, the harder it is to secure positions for residency training in the United States. Such observation is not totally unfounded and has led to some international medical graduates who graduated several years before arriving in the United States to consider alternative career options.

In our current effort with many still in medical school with a desire to travel to the United States for postgraduate medical training, we now recommend that they start making plans during the last three years of their study. Such an approach not only encourages such students to focus on their studies, but also to apply their current knowledge in taking the appropriate qualifying examinations while they are resident outside of the United States.

Unless your medical school is not accredited for the purpose of postgraduate training in the United States, there is no point in traveling to the United

States before taking the early components of the qualifying examinations. It also eliminates the expenses associated with travel and living in the United States without any guarantee of employment.

****

I did not hear back from Adeshua over a period of three months, although I kept her name and email address on my active follow-up list to check on at some point in time. When I finally heard back from her, it was in the form of an actual letter mailed to my office. It was obvious she had obtained my office address from an earlier communication. In the letter was a copy of a receipt of her payment to sit a component of the United States Medical Licensing Examination USMLE, due to be completed later in the year. Included in the envelope, was a postcard that read:

'Dear Sir, I am moving ahead with my plan to immigrate to the United States. I am due to sit my test as you can see (document attached), and I am currently studying towards it. Do you have any tips on when to apply for a travel visa? Yours truly. Adeshua.'

I don't often get such communications in the form of an actual letter. In fact as at the time I received that letter, I had not received any such letters in the prior two years, an understandable fact, with the popularity of emails and broadband Internet access to many countries. Not only was the means of communication uncommon, the question raised was quite unusual. It was obvious that Adeshua has no specific destination in mind, even though she has a plan to travel. Since I was no expert at immigration law, I was very careful in my response.

'Dear Adeshua, I am glad to learn that you would soon be taking the USMLE examination. I hope you are putting your best effort into the preparation. With respect to your question, there is no perfect time to apply for a visa, although unless you plan to travel just for vacation, it may be a little premature. I would recommend that you focus on passing the first two stages of your examinations and defer any unrelated travel until later. The following websites will be of relevance as you think ahead in your travel plan:

- *http://travel.state.gov/content/visas/english.html*
- *https://ceac.state.gov/genniv/*
- *http://nigeria.usembassy.gov/non-immigrant_visas.html*

Regards'

TIPS/LESSONS

While I see the reasoning behind Adeshua's plan in terms of applying for a travel visa early, I was concerned that applying for a visa at that point in time may be a distraction. Unless you are well to do, and have a lot of time and money at your disposal, it may not be a good idea altogether. It is also important to remember that there is no guarantee that a visa application will be successful at your first attempt. Such an untoward outcome may be a source of discouragement at a time when you need to focus more on your studies.

While it is important to obtain a travel visa, I think it is even more important to know what part of the United States you plan to visit, and what the purpose of your journey is. Are you going there for a vacation? If so, how long do you plan to stay for?

It is very important to think through your long-term goal and the travel visa requirement as it applies to your circumstance. What you do not want to do is to be in too much of a hurry to enter the United States that you fail to think through your options in terms of the various immigration visa requirements.

****

After my last communication with Adeshua, I received emails from her at roughly monthly interval, with updates on her the progress with her study preparation. Through one of such emails, I learned she had completed her National Youth Service posting and went on to work at a small hospital in a remote village in the Northern part of Nigeria. I also learned that because she was one of the two doctors available at the hospital, she did not have enough time to engage in her study preparation. When she sat for the examination the first time, she failed, and she almost gave up on her plan to travel. Her communication at that time showed the state of her mind after failing the test. It was a much shorter email that the ones I had received in the past.

'Dear Sir, I recently got my test results. It was not good. I know my work schedule was the problem as I am constantly on-call, and I could barely study after work. I think I might have to abandon my travel plans for now. I thank you for your support so far. Yours truly, Adeshua.'

When I received this particular email, it was forwarded to my assistant immediately for attention the next time we were scheduled to meet. That was two days later. Instead of sending another email in reply, I remembered that she had written her telephone number on the postcard she had mailed to me some months earlier. That afternoon after my clinic session, I called the number to talk directly to her. She was not available at the time, but I was able to leave her a voicemail message. About three hours later, my phone rang and I recognized the number I had called earlier. Our conversation was very short when I talked to her.

"It's me Adeshua."

"I saw your email and know exactly what you are going through. I went through an experience not dissimilar to what you have just shared with me. My prescription to your problem is to leave the job and find one that allows you to study, or not work at all until you sit and pass your tests."

"I'm not sure I can do that," was the response from her.

"Then you are not ready to come to the United States," I said bluntly.

At that point, the telephone line went dead. I was not sure if it was the result of a poor connection, or whether she ran out of prepaid telephone minutes, a common billing practice among mobile phone users in Nigeria. As I thought about our conversation later that evening, I wondered if my approach was too blunt and unfriendly. I however felt there was no better way to make an impact at such critical time.

I did not hear back from Adeshua for several months. In fact I had written her off as one of those who had the desire but lacked the will, until I received another letter in the mail with the result of her test scores enclosed. Hers was the last letter I was expecting. Not only did she pass the test, she scored at the upper level of performance. In the postcard that accompanied the letter, she wrote:

'Dear Sir, I did as you prescribed. It worked as you predicted. I will await your recommendation on my visa application. Yours truly, Adeshua.'

I felt it was time to make up for my bluntness the last time I spoke to her. I passed her information to my assistant who continued to talk to her and guide her through the visa application process. She was able to get the necessary documents in support of her travel visa application, and connect her with a host family in Elizabeth, New Jersey, where she stayed while she completed the remaining components of the USMLE and applied for a residency training position.

TIPS/LESSONS

While your story might be different in details when compared to that of Adeshua, it is not too far off from that of many immigrants who are now live in the United States. Many have had to go through such steps, some with greater difficulties. It is important to know that certain decisions will have to be made by you, and you alone, to fulfill your dream of coming to the United States. It's what we call sacrifice, which comes in many forms: time, money, effort, diligence, and focus. Without these sacrifice, your desire will remain a dream.

The following is a list of pathways through which international medical graduates have entered the United States in the past, prior to obtaining positions for residency training:

- Securing a postgraduate Masters degree - MPH, MBA or PhD programs
- Obtaining positions as a research assistant
- Getting a clinical, or non-clinical fellowship, or clerkship

Except for individuals who were born in the United States, and those married to United States citizens and the few that were fortunate to have won the immigrant visa lottery, you will need to pass through one of these pathways to legally reside in the United States. All of these alternatives provide opportunities to pursue additional postgraduate studies and/or research prior to starting a residency program.

Another important question that comes to mind in this story is the issue of National Youth Service, an obligation that every graduate from Nigerian Colleges of Higher Education have to complete before joining the workforce. While I am a proponent for you completing the yearlong obligation to your country, it may not be relevant if you do not intend to return to the country to practice in the immediate future. It may also add to your number of years post-graduation when you are being considered for residency training interviews. That year may be better put to use studying for the necessary examinations towards your postgraduate training. This same reasoning applies to those who plan to pursue a portion of their postgraduate training in their country of graduation before crossing over to the United States. It may be a worthwhile endeavor while you are waiting to get the opportunity to travel. For those who plan to return to their country of origin following completion of postgraduate training in the United States, there is always an opportunity to do so at a later date.

LIVING IN AMERICA – HOW DO I SURVIVE?

The subject of this chapter plays hand-in-hand with the one that was discussed in the earlier chapter. It is a reality that dawn on many sooner than anticipated as the time to embark on the journey to the United States approaches. The intricacies of this question will be demonstrated in the form of another short story.

While on call at a local hospital eighteen miles south of Boston early one morning, I received a telephone call from a colleague about an international medical graduate who had arrived a few days earlier from Ghana with a group of tourists to visit the historical landmarks in Washington, D.C. He had decided at the last minute to extend his stay and explore the options for continuing his medical education in the United States. His name was Sam. My friend invited me to a meeting with Sam at a local bakery very early the next day.

We met the following morning as planned, at a nondescript bakery tucked behind an auto repair shop in Quincy, Massachusetts. After a brief introduction, I ordered a plain bagel and cream cheese, before settling down on a cold metal chair.

Prior to his arrival in Boston, he had contacted a distant cousin, a married woman, who worked at a local hotel as a manager. Even though it was unclear what transpired in the conversation between the two of them, his version was that the woman would offer him temporary accommodation pending the time he found his footing. Unfortunately for him, when he arrived in Boston, he found out that the telephone number provided by the woman had been disconnected. Attempts to track his cousin down were unsuccessful, leaving with the option to stay in a motel on the outskirt of town.

After a few nights at the motel, he took the unusual step of visiting one of the big hospitals in Boston to look for assistance. It was there that he ran into taxi cab driver that had come to drop a patient at the hospital. It was the taxi driver that made the connection to my friend.

TIPS/LESSONS

While the experience shared in the story is unusual, it is not an uncommon occurrence. It continues to surprise me why some people would arrive into the United States and expect to be housed by some relative they had spoken to in years. It was not a surprise that Sam's cousin did what she did, although it is difficult to justify such an action to someone coming to from West Africa where the expectations might be different. The lessons in this story are many; the first one is that you obtain a real confirmation from a host, or hostess before you make your journey. The second lesson is that you should always have an alternative option when you plan your trip to the United States. Even if Sam's cousin was really willing to assist, anything could have happened between when they both communicated, and when he eventually arrive in the country.

The challenge with Sam's story extends beyond where to stay, but also include the one question that many often hesitate to talk about, especially to someone they don't really know. This subject is covered in the continuation of this story.

While I ate my bagel and crème cheese, Sam had a couple of croissants, while my friend only had a cup of coffee, claiming he hardly eats breakfast. He was the one that broached the subject of immigration.

"Are you on a visiting visa?" he asked.

"Kind of," Sam replied, after a moment of hesitance that tells me he was not sure whether I should be privy to such information.

"How long do you plan to stay?" I asked to confirm my earlier assumption.

"Until I can finally settle down," he replied.

I looked at my friend who sat just across the table and covertly winked at him as Sam talked.

"You know that may take forever if you don't have the right visa?" my friend asked.

"I am hoping there will be a way to make my visa right," he finally said.

"Yes, there sure is," I said with a chuckle. "Which one do you know about?"

He looked at me with narrowed eyes, as if I had stuck a pin in the back of his hand. It was apparent he has no immediate answers, or if he did, he was not willing to let me know of his plans. My friend got the message more than I did.

"Don't even bother, my friend interjected, before Sam could voice what he has on his mind. I will send him to the immigration lawyer that lives next door to me," he added.

With the discussion on immigration laid to rest, at least temporarily, we were able to address the issue of housing, at least in the short term. While still at the table, we both made some phone calls to a couple of friends that we know in our community. We found success much quicker than we had anticipated, as we were able to get a local church that would offer temporary housing for a period of four weeks. It was all we needed, at least, until we can make a more concrete arrangement. We adjourned our meeting with a plan to meet in three days and continue our discussion where we left it.

I offered to take him back to his hotel where he was able to pick up his personal belongings, and then drive him to the church where we both met the clergy in charge. Sam looked in disbelief, and was mute for the rest of the morning as he was overwhelmed by the speed with which we had both come to his assistance. I waived at him as a volunteer at the church led him away down a stairway into the basement of the church.

TIPS/LESSONS

When I counsel individuals that are in the country for the first time, I am always direct in my discussions with them. I make it my business to know as much as I could in the short time I have to meet them; not only about their medical school and experience to date, but their family, their aspirations and goals. The issue of immigrations ranks high in my list of questions, as it makes no sense to invest time in mentoring an individual only to be told later that the person has overstayed their immigration visa. Knowing the answer to that single question also helps in how one directs his, or her effort in your role as an advisor. Generally, I let those who are experts at immigration deal with the issue of visa requirement, while I play the role I am comfortable with during the process. The next part of this story highlights other important aspects of living in the United States.

****

The next time we met, my friend was unable to attend, due to the constraints of work. The fact that there were just the two of us present, allowed for a more engaging discussion. It was in the month of June and the weather was warm and friendly. This time, we met in front of the Boston Public library. Rather than sitting inside the library to have our discussion, we selected a quiet corner on the set of steps that line the northern wing of the building. We had to wait for a young man on a skating board to finish his maneuver before we could finally sit down.

"What have you been up to?" I asked, once we settled down.

"I have spent the last two days learning about Boston. It's the only city in America that I had wanted to visit, and possibly live in since I was in high school," he replied. He went on to tell me how much he had done over the last few days.

I was impressed by how much Sam had learnt about the City of Boston, in the short time that he was there – its history and tradition, the people, the local medical institutions and its geography. He was also able to register at the library and borrow books to do with the preparatory examinations towards his goal to further his medical training.

"I'm impressed." It was all I could say by the time he was done telling me all he had accomplished in a short time.

He had also met with an immigration lawyer the day before. He described the meeting as helpful and productive, and he seemed to have learnt so much on the options available to him, that he was able to school me on the current developments on immigration. Sam was very fortunate that he had another five months left on his travel visa before it would expire, giving him the time to explore the various avenues to extend his time if he so desires.

TIPS/LESSONS

The lesson from this section of the story centers on how what you achieve is dependent on your effort and your attitude. In the earlier part of this story, you saw how Sam took the unusual step of visiting a local hospital in the hope of meeting a helper. It worked in his case, and for those who try, the outcome could only be one of two possibilities – success, or failure. In other words, you should be prepared to take meaningful, but bold actions in your quest to achieve your goals.

The same aggression was demonstrated in how he sought out information pertaining to his primary goal of pursuing postgraduate training in the United States. While it is unique in the case of Sam that he was drawn to Boston since his high school days, and understanding that such intense desire had influenced his energy and focus, we can learn some lessons from this story. With the plethora of information on the Internet, it is now possible to attain many of these feats in the comfort of your house, well before you even place your feet on the American soil.

The central theme in this discourse is the significance of connecting with whatever part of the country you find yourself. Not only should you be concerned about those things that relate directly to your career, also find out about people that you may know, like classmates, family friends, or a community of people from your part of the world. I often get people referred to me by a good friend of mine who runs a multi-service store; on some other occasions, it is from a nurse that works at the local hospital where I consult. Getting to know people and finding out very early is vital, especially if you do not have anyone, as it is in the case of Sam. These people will have tangible

information, particularly those that does not feature on the Internet that may end up shaping the course of your life. The next part of this story tells what path Sam took and the other challenges he ran into as he tried to settle down.
****
****

After I had listened to Sam talk endlessly about what he already know about Boston and surrounding towns, I asked him how much money he has with him, and whether it would last the five months that he has before his travel visa expires.

"Money to spend?" he asked, putting his right hand in the front pocket of his pant, as if he was about to pull out a wad of dollars. When he pulled his hand out, it was empty.

"Unhuh," I replied, curtailing myself no to laugh and cause any embarrassment.

"To be frank, I have one hundred and forty dollars and seventy cent left."

I kept a neutral face and wondered at what rate he would burn through the amount of money he has just declared he had in his possession. It seemed very unlikely that it would last that much.

"How much do you spend per day?"

"Nothing, since you helped me to find a place to stay at the church. They serve breakfast after morning prayers, and they do the same after evening worship, so I make sure I attend the two services. I also keep enough bread rolls saved up from breakfast in my bag to eat during the day."

He saw the look on my face after and smiled. I could tell he is very resourceful, but I was not sure the amount of money he has would get him through the next five months.

Before the end of the meeting, we set up another meeting to discuss and formulate a path that would yield the best outcome.

TIPS/LESSONS

From the meeting, one could easily deduce the priorities. Some of these are listed:

- To make the most of his remaining five months in the United States
- To decide on which of the examinations to take before living
- To explore the opportunity of acquiring clinical skills locally
- To consider alternative sources of funding for the rest of his stay

Our next meeting was very brief, with Sam arriving at my office for the meeting. The possible challenges were discussed at length, and the possibilities were considered, before finally settling on the most attractive solution. At this meeting, I also discovered that his travel visa is a multiple entry visa type that allows him to return to the United States on two or three more occasions. It was a great relief, one that offered the flexibility to approach the challenges differently.

Sam was advised to take the Clinical Skills component of the examination while he was still in the United States, since it is the one examination that requires physical presence in the United States. With the next session of the Clinical Skills examination not due for another three months, Sam had the option to return to Ghana before both his funds and visa run out.

While he was preparing for the Clinical Skills examination, he secured a six-week observership position to brush up his clinical skills. With respect to the issue of housing and lack of funds, he was able to work out a deal with the local church to extend his offer of free accommodation to three and a half month, complimentary breakfast and dinner, in return for his service to tend the church's ground.

TIPS/LESSONS

Not many cases are as complicated as it was made to be in the last story. More and more people are getting better prepared, with improved knowledge of the living requirements, and with enough money to last through the early stages of their stay.

It will be a good exercise to consider the alternatives that are available to someone in Sam's situation, had he not had the opportunity of a multiple entry travel visa that allows him to leave and return to the United States at a later date. Many international medical graduates use the opportunity of the first visit to the country to secure university admissions for non-clinical postgraduate studies, and as such are able to change their immigration visa type to one that is applicable to international students. This option is not available to everyone since the question of the cost of the education becomes relevant. It is still possible to secure such postgraduate study positions based on the offer of a scholarship, or with the offer of a university-backed education loan.

Other alternative includes looking for a research position that guarantees change of immigration visa status. Additional information on the various immigration visa options can be obtained from a qualified immigration attorney.

The solution provided with respect to housing in this case is not achievable in most circumstances. A more reliable approach will be to obtain a listing of accommodations available for short-term rental. Some of the rentals consist of single rooms, which are more affordable than self-contained units. Such lists are readily available over the Internet using appropriate search keywords. The farther out you are from the cities in general, the less expensive the rental rate becomes, although someone must be prepared to face the challenge of transportation.

Other aspects of life include transportation – taxis, buses, trains, and commuter rails, and in some instances, the need to obtain a driver's license. Relevant websites on the subject of transportation specific to the Boston area can be obtained from the following websites:

http://www.mbta.com/
http://www.massrmv.com/

Access to medical services is an important aspect of living in the United States that many often be ignored until the last moment. It is advisable to register with local health centers, as they offer easier access, and are less expensive alternatives to using the emergency rooms of tertiary hospitals. The services available at these centers cover an array of medical specialties, including dental and social services. For a listing of local health centers in your area, visit the following website:

http://nachc.com/default.cfm

The Examination Maze – What is there to know?

There are so many stories around the subject of preparation and registration for the required examinations in order to embark on medical residency training in the United States. Some of these stories center on when to sit for the examination and the order in which one should sit the examination, while many more center on how best to prepare for the examination. Other questions I personally have had to deal with include whether getting a residency position depends solely on your performance in the examinations, and whether a less impressive score is equivalent to a zero chance of securing a medical residency position.

As the aspect of your preparation for the examination is very important, I will dedicate this chapter and the next to explore the various scenarios based on past experiences and help you, the reader to determine which approach works best for you.

The format of the examination is very straightforward, as outlined in the booklet available from the examination body responsible for setting up and administering the various examinations. This information is readily available on the Internet on the following websites:

- http://www.usmle.org/
- http://www.fsmb.org/
- http://www.nbme.org/
- http://ecfmg.org/

These websites are most likely to provide you with updates on changes with the examinations, especially those that relate to the formats and the schedules.

The USMLE website not only provide you adequate information – content and description, it offers you downloadable practice questions, tutorials and videos at no cost to the examinee. These resources are of immense benefit in your preparation effort towards the examinations. Regular visits to these websites is particularly helpful to keep you abreast of scheduled changes, as this may be critical if you have a tight schedule ahead of you and you plan to applying for a residency position in the same year that your are sitting the examination.

The NBME website offers a portal that enables an examinee to complete a pre-examination assessment of your competency at a cost. While the cost to complete such pre-assessment tests may be an issue to some, it is an additional resource that provides you with an objective way to assess your readiness. This is not necessary in all cases, as I have come across international medical graduates that did very well without using this resource.

In additional to the information available through the examining bodies, there are several commercial sources of information pertaining to preparation towards examination. It remains unclear whether the money spent on such additional resources is money well spent, as there are many that vouch for their value, as there are many that wished they had never bought such services. My advice is that you keep talking to those who have gone ahead of you, hoping that they will be generous enough to share their experiences with you, and save you from making the same mistakes. Irrespective of the path that you decide to take, never believe any of the claims made by such entities in its entirety, as they are primarily motivated to sell you their services.

While every effort has been made to ensure that the information provided in this chapter is not exactly what you would obtain on the examining bodies websites, it is still important to cover the basic aspects of the various examinations.

The purpose of this chapter and the next is not to offer you, the reader, a guarantee of success in your examination, but to offer you guidance on the questions often asked in the preparation towards the examination. In the chapter that follows this chapter, I will address the subject of how best to prepare for the examination, and give an insight into how to best utilize the resources at your disposal.

What are the various components of the United States Medical Licensing Examination (USMLE)?

The following is a list of the of the United States Medical Licensing Examination (USMLE):

- Step 1
- Step 2, CK (Clinical Knowledge)
- Step 2 CS (Clinical Skills)
- Step 3

It is important to note that Step 1, Step 2 CS, or Step 2 CK may be taken in any sequence once you meet the eligibility criteria. Step 3 is the only step of the examinations that may not be completed until the other steps are fully completed.

What are the requirements to participate in the various components of the examination?

- Step 1
  - Enrollment in a medical school that is listed in IMED (International Medical Education Directory) and meet the eligibility criteria of the ECFMG (Educational Commission for Foreign Medical Graduates).
- Step 2 CK
  - Enrollment in a medical school that is listed in IMED (International Medical Education Directory) and meet the eligibility criteria of the ECFMG (Educational Commission for Foreign Medical Graduates).
- Step 2 CS
  - Enrollment in a medical school that is listed in IMED (International Medical Education Directory) and meet the eligibility criteria of the

ECFMG (Educational Commission for Foreign Medical Graduates).

- Entry into the United States, as the test is conducted within the United States.

- Step 3

  - Success at Step 1, Step 2 CS and 2 CK, with not more than six attempts.

  - Completion of an MD, or DO degree, or equivalent qualification from a medical school that is listed in IMED (International Medical Education Directory) and meet the eligibility criteria of the ECFMG (Educational Commission for Foreign Medical Graduates).

  - ECFMG certification, or successfully complete the 'Fifth Pathway'.

What is the minimum passing score for the different stages of the examination?

- Step 1
  - 192
- Step 2 CK
  - 209
- Step 2 CS
  - Pass/Fail
- Step 3
  - 190

When is the best time to sit for the various examinations?

- Step 1
  - It used to be that many international graduates sit the examination after graduation from medical school, the trend

nowadays, especially if you already plan to leave the country for postgraduate medical training, is to sit this stage of the examination while still at medical school, a time when your knowledge base of the basic science curriculum is still fresh. The medical students in the United States tend to take Step 1 on completion of the second year of medical school, while Step 2 is generally completed in the final year. When you take Step 1 matters with respect to when you plan to take Step 3, as the State Licensing bodies make it a requirement all the steps of the USMLE are completed within a period of seven years, with the exception of MD/PhD candidates who may be given an exemption under the right circumstances to complete the steps of the examination within a period of nine years.

- Step 2

  - When you sit this stage of the examination depends on a

number of factors. You do not need to sit Step 1 examination before sitting any of the components of Step 2. In the case of Step 2 CS, you need to be physically present in the United States to sit this component of the examination. More importantly, the timing of your participation in the examination should depend on your preparedness, and on the time you plan to apply to residency training programs, and participate in the Match. In other words, you need to be done taking the required components of the examination in such time that your test scores will be available for consideration with the rest of your application for the available residency positions.

Because of the rate at which the available spaces for completion of the two components of this examination fill up (over three to four months ahead of time), it is advisable to apply for the examination by May 31 of the calendar year in which you plan to sit the examination. This will also give you ample time to receive your examination scores and make them available for residency programs that you want to apply to for consideration.

- Step 3

  - While it is the norm to sit for this examination during your first year of residency training, a number of international medical graduates elect to sit the examination before they commence training. For many, the motivation for taking the examination before starting residency training is to make them more competitive while applying for residency programs, while for others, it is a way to put their time to great use while waiting to commence residency training.

    In my experience working with international medical graduates, when you decide to sit this stage of the examination is not that important, although some residency programs may consider it during the selection process for residency training. One clear advantage is the fact that it will make you eligible for full licensure with the State Board of Registration/Licensure well before you complete your residency training.

I have also heard from many that it may be of benefit when an international medical graduate secures residency training, and requires an immigration visa for training. Those who are of this opinion believe that they are more likely to obtain an H1-B visa, the type of visa that allows you stay on in the United States when you finally complete your residency training, as opposed to a J-1 visa that requires that you leave the United States for a specified number of years at the end of your residency training, before you can return to seek employment.

What is the format for the various examination stages?

- Step 1
  - This test is completed in one day.
  - The day consists of an 8-hour test session.
- Step 2
  - This test is completed within two non-consecutive days.
  - Each day consists of an 8-hour test session.
  - Day 1 of the examination consists of Clinical Knowledge (CK), mostly multiple-choice questions (MCQ).
  - Day 2 of the examination consists of Clinical Skills (CS), a 12-patient clinical encounter split into three sections of 5, 4, and 3 patients per session.
- Step 3
  - This test is completed over two days.

- Each day consists of an 8-hour test session.
- Day 1 of the examination consists of Foundations of Independent Practice (FIP), mostly multiple-choice questions (MCQ).
- Day 2 of the examination consists of Advanced Clinical Medicine (ACM), a combination of multiple-choice questions (MCQ) and computer base case simulations (CCS).

Why is it so expensive to sit these examinations?

This is a question that comes up all the time when I talk to international medical graduates, especially those who are still resident in their country of origin, and those who may not have the support of a family member. Not only is it expensive to sit the various components of the examination for all examinees, there is the added cost for the international medical graduate who is resident outside of the United States and Canada, in terms of the international delivery surcharge applicable to those examinations that can be completed outside of the United States and Canada. This is probably another reason why many wait for a few years following graduation, to work and be able to save some money.

Conducting examinations such as the United States Medical Licensing Examinations (USMLE) is not as easy as it seems, and do require a lot of resources to implement it successfully. Like everything else that is not open to market competition, the prices are likely to continue in line with inflation. While it is not in your power to influence the fees stipulated to register for these examinations, you can exercise control in how many times you give your money to the organizing bodies, by making sure you only participate in the examination when you know that you are fully ready, and when you believe you can pass and score highly in the examinations.

When you consider the added costs like travel, books purchases, and attendance at preparatory classes, it becomes clear that this is a major career investment, and one that is worth every effort that you can muster. If you plan to cancel, postpone, or reschedule an examination, it is important to do so well in advance, as there are additional cost to pay if it is done too close to the date of the examination. The same applies to a change of location for completing the examination, if it is not done within the stipulated time frame.

Why do I have to travel so far to take these examinations?

In talking about the cost involved in completing the various steps of the USMLE examination, one cannot ignore the cost that relates to travel and accommodation. If for example, you are located in Nigeria, you will find out that your test center is located in Accra, Ghana. Depending on where in Nigeria an examinee is located, that individual will have to make it to a major city in Nigeria, before embarking on the journey to Accra, Ghana.

Back to the main question of why you have to travel far to sit for the examinations, there are significant logistical requirements and security issues with respect to test materials that the organizing body have to deal with that is only possible to successfully operate a limited number of test centers. The spread of test centers in the West African subcontinent is more spread out, than one may observe in say, Europe, or other continents where there are longer established relationship for such examinations. A good knowledge of the examination centers in your region is very important prior to registering to take any step of the examinations.

A visit to this website - https://www.prometric.com - will tell you which examination centers are closest to your location of residence and the availability of spaces on your preferred date. It is also important to note that availability of test centers may change without notice for reasons best known to the examining bodies.

Can I retake failed examinations?

While this is a question one hope not to be seeking an answer for, it is not unreasonable to want to figure out what your options are well before you sit the examination. You can definitely retake failed examination, although there are set limitations on how many times you can retake a test in the space of twelve months. The USMLE website provides specific details on these limitations with respect to the various steps of the examination.

More importantly, you would want to know if the fact that you had to retake any step of the examination would count against you when you apply for residency positions. This latter question has no easy answer, as your ability to secure a position for residency training depends on other factors outside of your performance at any step of the examination.

Does failure to attend for an examination count as a failure?

This is a question that has come up several times in discussions with international medical graduates. The most current answer to this question can always be obtained at the USMLE website. The current practice is that incomplete attempt will count towards the number of times one has attempted a step of the examination. Failure to attend for a registered examination does not count as an attempt, or a failure. There are alternatives short of not attending for a registered examination, such as rescheduling, changing the location, or canceling, some of which may be associated with additional costs.

Can I retake passed examinations?

Generally, the answer to this question is no, although the USMLE guideline offer a rare instance when it may be allowed, as a condition to comply with the requirement of a State Licensing body.

This chapter will be incomplete without the short stories that characterized the first two chapters of this book. Like the narratives in the earlier chapters, this story is based on fictional characters, and serves the primary purpose of reinforcing the fact that despite the challenges that are often associated with completion of the various components of this examination, it is well possible to overcome the difficulties and make progress towards achieving your goals.

****

On my last trip to Nigeria, I was sitting with two sisters, who happen to be twins, named Bridget, the other named Helen. It was a totally accidental encounter, one that did not happen anywhere near the vicinity of an academic setting. I was visiting a local artisan in Oyo, a historical town, with a rich cultural heritage, and was admiring a wood carving of the bust of Hippocrates that had been commissioned by a customer, when the two of them turned up to collect it. Out of curiosity, I inquired why they had commissioned the work, and wondered why they would spend so much money on it. It was then that they announced that they are medical students, and that a group of students had contributed the money to make the purchase for a departing professor at their medical school, located in another town. It was then that I engaged them in a discussion around their field of study.

We talked about their medical school; their future plans following graduation, and the thought of traveling overseas for training. Throughout the conversation, I did not mention the fact that I was in the profession, although I made a cursory remark to the fact that I had a nephew that had traveled to the United States for postgraduate medical training. After a lengthy conversation, I advised them to inquire about traveling to the United States for postgraduate training. When they were leaving, I handed them my business card. It was then they realized that I was a physician visiting from the United States. I encouraged them to keep in touch and update me about their progress with their studies.

In subsequent communications over several months via email, I was kept abreast of their progress. In their first email, the sisters thanked me for the advice I had offered, and informed me that they had set out to pursue a component of the USMLE while still enrolled at medical school. Because of the cost of registering for the examination, it was impossible for the two of them to enroll at the same time. Since they had some time ahead of them in their planning, they came up with an arrangement enabled them to rotate their participation in the examination. The arrangement not only allowed them to save towards the examination fees, but rather than wait until they have both saved enough, they combined their savings, and had one sister register and sit the examination first, while the other waits, while they saved enough money for the other sister to apply for the test. The arrangement also allowed them to register for different components of the examination when it was the time of the individual to participate.

Helen was supposed to register first for the examination, taking Step 1, while Bridget was supposed to wait, and whenever it was her turn to register for the examination, to apply for Step 2 CK. The two of them did not start applying for the examinations until the fourth year of a six-year medical school program, although they had started studying much earlier. Helen was then allocated the task of completing the registration for the examinations for the two of them, as a result she had spent a significant amount of time on the USMLE website, learning all she could about the examination requirements and guidelines. Bridget on the other hand, focused on getting all the preparatory resources, such as testing materials, books, and practice questions textbooks.

Interestingly for the two sisters, they had decided to study for the two components of the examination at the same time, as they have always studied together for other examinations in their years together in high school and at medical school. It was an approach they had taken towards their studies over the years to help each other in their preparatory effort. They took turns to complete practice USMLE test questions for both the Step 1 and Step 2 CK during their period of study.

Some four to five months into their preparation, Helen went ahead with the registration process in accordance with the plan register one sister at a time. Rather than complete the registration process herself, she delegated the job to their father, a high school principal who had made a contribution to their savings and had kept the money meant for registration on their behalf. When their father proceeded with the registration process, unfortunately for them, instead of registering Helen first for the Step 1 component of the examination, he made the mistake of registering Bridget first. That was not the only mistake he made, instead of registering Bridget for the Step 2 CK component of the examination as planned, he registered her for the Step 1 component. The two sisters did not find out until a few weeks later, but early enough to make adjustment in the preparation plans and effort.

They both deliberated on whether to reschedule, or cancel the examination, as they were not only well advanced in their preparation for different components of the examination, the order of participation had been revised. Because of the cost associated with rescheduling the examination at that stage of the preparation, and since they had studied concurrently for the two components of the examination, rather than incur any additional costs associated with such changes, it was agreed that Bridget would go ahead and sit the Step 1 of the examination. Even though the mistake and the forced change in plan was a cause of stress and tension at a time when they needed none, Bridget proceeded to sit for Step 1 component of the examination and excelled. Helen then waited for her turn to take the Step 1 of the examination. They both then waited until they have saved enough money to sit the Step 2 CK test together, and did so successfully. With respect to their father, and his unforgettable mistake, it was the last time the two sisters would delegate such duties to him.

TIPS/LESSONS

Like many stories that you would come across in this book, they often look very real, and as it is when mistakes do happen, one always think it can never happen to them. There are many lessons to learn from Bridget and Helen - their dedication, and the ingenuity in combining resources at a time when individually it would have been impossible. It however does require a significant amount of trust and loyalty to implement such a strategy with someone that is not a family member. There is something to learn in their approach to study, a subject that I will touch on in the next chapter of this book. While this story is unique and may not be the norm, it highlights the possible sources of errors.

The Examination Hurdle – How do I best prepare?

The title of this chapter is a reminder of a personal experience during my preparation for the PLAB examination, the British equivalent of the USMLE. It was in the late 80's and I was part of a group of international medical graduates who had come from Nigeria to London, England to sit for the test. At the time, there were rumors that the success rate for the PLAB examination was very discouraging, none of which we had no way of confirming. The majority of the people in that group had graduated around the same year and most of us came from the same medical school. Rather than worry about the rumors of how people were failing the tests, we set out to find those who have passed the test to learn about their experiences. It was not that difficult to find those who had passed the test, as we all studied at a local hospital's library – Whittington Hospital in Archway, Islington, North London. There we met a few international medical graduates and talked to them about what they attributed to their success. A few of the individuals in our group were also able to find out about a couple of alumni that had passed the tests and asked them the same questions.

The common theme that we discovered with the ones that passed the test was the way they prepared for the examination. Not a single one of them studied in isolation during the time of preparation. Instead, they were part of a group of four to six individuals that stayed together right from the moment they register for the test to when they pass and moved on to the next stage of their career. In those individuals that studied together, the success rate was over 75 percent. Even though our group at the time was based on the fact that we had arrived in the country around the same time, and had attended the same medical school, we quickly turned the group to a study group. The group was a little larger than the ones we had understudied, as an additional two international medical graduates were invited to join. In all, there were about nine of us in the group. We all completed our individual studies in the morning, most of the times using the hospital's library, and at about four-thirty in the afternoon, would meet at the hospital's cafeteria for a study group session. The sessions usually lasted about ninety minutes, followed by a dinner at the cafeteria during which the discussion continues in a less formal setting, before we depart for our various destinations. Over a course of six months, we all religiously followed this routine, with every one of us committed and encouraging each other throughout the process. We all sat the examination together, and nine of the ten of us in the group passed at the first attempt, the one person that did not succeed, did so at the second attempt.

TIPS/LESSONS

There is no set way to prepare for an examination like the USMLE. So much of how you prepare depends on your individual style in terms of studying. Not many international medical graduates will have the luxury of a small group like the one referenced in the story I had just narrated. Unless you are in a major academic city like Boston, New York, or Chicago, you may never find that many people studying for the same examination about the same time. Some of the components of the USMLE examinations do not lend themselves as well to a group study approach. While the majority of your knowledge acquisition is through individual effort, reinforcement of knowledge sometimes occurs in the discussions that take place in a group. The obvious benefit of this approach is the one that relates to an increase in your knowledge base. Of greater value is the comfort that one gains knowing that you are not alone in your journey, and the confidence that develops as you get the opportunity to gauge your preparedness against your peers.

Every group has something unique that they impart on its participant, depending on the people involved, and the prevailing circumstances in their lives. This approach will not work for everybody, although it is worthwhile considering if you have never experienced it before.

The next segment of this chapter will be devoted to a discussion on the experiences of four candidates who had completed different components of the United States Medical Licensing Examination (USMLE). As you follow the transcripts of the interviews of these candidates, you will find aspects that will be of benefit in your preparation.

Interview #1

This is a transcript of an interview I had with J.Z, an international medical graduate who recently passed Step 1 of the United States Medical Licensing Examination (USMLE).

Dr. O': Congratulations J.Z.! Heard you aced your Step 1. What was your score?

J.Z: Thanks. I scored 256.

Dr. O': Great stuff! I am happy for you.

J.Z: I thank you for your support.

Dr. O': That's not bad after just three months of study.

J.Z: I wish it were three months. It was much closer to six months.

Dr. O′: Really? Could you have done it in three months?

J.Z: I don't know about that. I believe that in my case, taking my time was very helpful.

Dr. O′: I bet you could do it in three months if you try.

J.Z: In retrospect, may be. It really depends on the individual. I have a friend that prepared for this stage of the examination for twelve months and scored 250; my other friend did it in three months and scored 236.

Dr. O′: Did you participate in any group study in your preparation, or did you limit yourself to self-study?

J.Z: I did both. I went through the Q bank with two other friends. In fact I went through it twice.

Dr. O′: What other resources did you use?

J.Z: I used First Aid, that book is a must have for the step 1. I read through it twice while answering questions using the U World Q bank. You may not fully appreciate the full potential of the book until you solve some questions using the U World Q bank. I also watched a few Kaplan videos on topics I wasn't too comfortable with, and completed three sessions of the NBME.

Dr. O': How many hours per day did you commit to reading?

J.Z: A minimum of 12 hours per day.

Dr. O': That's a lot of hours per day. Didn't you have to work?

J.Z: You are not the first to say so, but I could not afford not to pass the test. I was fortunate that I did not have to work in that period as I lived rent-free at my aunt's apartment.

Dr. O': Where did you complete most of your reading?

J.Z: I practically lived in the library for the duration of my preparation. I was in the library Monday to Friday from nine in the morning till it closed at night. On weekends, I put in extra hours of study at night. There were few days when I wasn't in the reading mood. On such days, the videos came in handy.

Dr. O': What can you say about the examination? Is it an easy test?

J.Z: The test is designed for people to pass, but it takes lots and lots of reading. Step 1 component of the examination is essentially the basics of Medicine - Anatomy, Biochemistry, Physiology and Pathology. These are subjects that form the bulk of the test. It is much harder to build up your knowledge base if it's been many years since you studied those subjects in medical school. In my case, that was over six years ago.

Dr. O': Was the eight hours allotted for the examination enough for you?

J.Z: Hmmm, that is a big question. Time is your enemy at the examination, I must say. You really don't have any time to waste on a question. You just need to have an idea, if not, just move to the next question. You may be lucky to have spare time to go back to those questions you were unsure of.

Dr. O': Did you have to guess while answering any of the questions?

J.Z: Yes, to a reasonable extent- educative guesses I will say. I tried to keep that to a minimum. I would rather skip the questions I do not have a good understanding of, than it waste any time.

Dr. O': How did you deal with the issue of fatigue on the examination day?

J.Z: I made sure I had quality rest a day prior to the examination. I had a light breakfast on the morning of the test.

Dr. O': Did anything change in your studying habit in the few days prior to the examination?

J.Z.: I spent a lot of time on the simulated examination questions. Throughout the day prior to the examination, I practiced the Q bank questions in an eight-hour stretch, doing the questions on multiple occasions.

Dr. O': Did you have any problem registering, or scheduling the examination?

J.Z: Not at all, it was without any hassle.

Dr. O': So how will you describe your overall strategy? Which parts of your preparation paid off?

J.Z: I will attribute my performance to my diligence and the consistency in my study effort. As soon as I made up my mind that I would take the examination, I set out with a mission to score high. I set it as a personal goal to study at least twelve hours a day, and resisted the temptation to work in the six months preceding the examination. I cut out all usual distractions, like web browsing, and unnecessary telephone calls.

Dr. O': I have a meeting coming up with a couple of international graduates. What advice should I give them with respect to preparing for the Step 1 of the United States Medical Licensing Examination (USMLE)?

J.Z: They must read extensively. 'First Aid' is a must have. U world Q bank is very essential. NBME will definitely help you to assess how well prepared you are for the examination. If your performance on the NBME test is unsatisfactory, I will recommend that you delay sitting the Step 1 of the United States Medical Licensing Examination (USMLE)

Dr. O': Thanks. I wish you well in your next examination.

J.Z: My pleasure.

Interview #2

This is another transcript of an interview I had with A.K, an international medical graduate after passing Step 2 CK component of the United States Medical Licensing Examination (USMLE).

Dr. O': Congratulations on passing Step 2.

A.K: Thanks.

Dr. O': It must be a relief to get through with this stage of the examination.

A.K: It's a big relief. I am so glad it's over.

Dr. O': Can you share your experience with me on how you studied for the test?

A.K: I would love to.

Dr. O': What resources did you use?

A.K: In my study effort, I used 'Step up to Medicine for Internal Medicine'. It was very helpful, as Internal Medicine constitute two-thirds of this component of the examination.

Dr. O': That's interesting.

A.K: I went through the whole volume of the book multiple times.

Dr. O': Any other resource?

A.K: I relied on Master the Boards for Step 2 CK - a great resource for reviewing the tips on questions that you would encounter in the examination.

Dr. O': What about practice questions?

A.K: Following the first three months of preparation for the examination, I completed U World Q bank questions religiously. I not only studied the way the questions are asked, but read the explanation that follows each answer. I also made sure I set the Q bank questions in timed mode during my preparation.

Dr. O': How important is that?

A.K: Very important, especially for timing your performance.

Dr. O': That seems to be a lot of work.

A.K: It is, but you've got to give it what it takes.

Dr. O': Any other tricks outside of what you already shared with me?

A.K: Nothing that comes immediately to mind.

Dr. O': What is your overall experience with the test?

A.K: Looking back, allocation of time during the actual test is very important. Step 2 CK is incredibly long - 9 hours in total. The fatigue you will experience is indescribable, and the best tip I can offer here is to practice ahead of time to build up your stamina.

Dr. O': Is there any important aspect of this test that we have not covered?

A.K: One more thing, you can take your preparation even further by completing a Kaplan simulated test. I took the simulated examination two weeks before the test day.

Dr. O': Did you engage in discussion groups during your preparation?

A.K: I relied more on personal study effort for this step of the examination. I also completed one month of clinical observership prior to sitting the examination. That opportunity allowed me to observe the management of many of the cases that came up in the examination.

Dr. O′: Was sitting other steps of the USMLE prior to your writing your Step 2 CK helpful?

A.K: Definitely. I completed Step 1 before embarking on the preparation for Step 2 CK.

Dr. O′: How did it help?

A.K: Studying for Step 1 of the examination refreshed my understanding of the basics of Medicine. In my case, it made studying Step 2 CK much easier and gave a better understanding of the management of diseases.

Dr. O′: What kind of questions did you see at the examination.

A.K: The questions have a general pattern. The formats are as listed:

- What is the most likely diagnosis?
- Which is the most appropriate initial step in management?
- Which of the following is the most appropriate next step in management?
- Which of the following is the most likely cause?
- Which of the following is the most likely pathogen?

In general, Internal Medicine constitutes two-third of the examination.

Dr. O': How long did you wait to get your result?

A.K: Three weeks.

Dr. O': Any other tip that you would like to offer?

A.K: Noting much more to add, although I must say that I was determined to do really well in my Step 2 CK examination since my Step 1 was not so good.

Interview #3

This is a transcript of an interview I had with B.J, an international medical graduate who recently passed Step 2 CS of the United States Medical Licensing Examination (USMLE).

Dr. O'- Well done B.J. I heard you did well in the Step 2 CS examination.

B.J.: Thank you, sir.

Dr. O': What resources did you use for your study?

B.J: I used 'First Aid – CS'. I found it adequate enough in my preparation, although I also utilized ' USMLE World cases'. I found significant overlap between the two. Kaplan is also a useful alternative that gives the opportunity of step-by-step practice on history-taking skill and clinical assessment.

Dr. O': Is there any strategy, or guideline that you followed in your preparation?

B.J: The key to this component of the examination is practice, practice, and practice. Having a basic knowledge of disease conditions in terms of their physiology and pathology is a requirement to doing well in this component of the examination.

Dr. O': What aspects of the examination did you actually focus on?

B.J: I familiarized myself with the kind of questions I should ask while taking a history from a patient. I worked on focused examination of a patient system by system. I also work on coming up with the differential diagnoses and the necessary work-ups to establish an actual diagnosis.

Dr. O': What else did you gain from your study practice?

B.J: I was able to improve my self-confidence, and my history-taking skills. I was able to improve my clinical documentation skills, and prepare better for difficult cases that may come up during the examination.

Dr. O': I understand that ones typing proficiency could be an issue in taking the examination. Did you find it so?

B.J: At the start of my study preparation, it was an issue.

Dr. O': How did you overcome the challenge?

B.J: This is an area where practice, practice, and practice worked. As an international medical graduate, I was not used to electronic medical records and typing patient notes on a computer back in medical school. What I did was to type at least five patient notes daily, until I was able to meet the allotted time of 10 minutes per case. In fact I got my pace down to 7 minutes by the time I was ready for the examination, leaving me 3 minutes to review my work. There are samples of standardized patient's clinical notes online that one can use to practice and improve ones typing skills.

Dr. O': Do you have any other suggestions on the subject of typing skills and performance in the examination?

B.J: It is also very helpful to familiarize oneself with the various standardized US abbreviations that are acceptable during the examination. It is another trick that can improve your speed of documentation.

Dr. O': How long did you practice for?

B.J: In total, I practiced over a period of four weeks, completing 5 cases per day.

Dr. O': How long did it take for the examination result to be released?

B.J: On the average, three months, with a slight variation in the timing.

Dr. O': Did you use a practice partner for this component of the examination?

B.J: Yes, of course. I doubt if I would have passed the examination that easily, and at the first attempt, without having a practice partner to discuss and review cases with.

Dr. O': Is your practice partner another international medical graduate like yours?

B.J: Not at all, I had a friend who relied on her roommate in a profession unrelated to Medicine, although it is much better if you practice with someone preparing for the examination like yourself.

Dr. O': Was it difficult for you to get a partner to practice with?

B.J: In my case, it was difficult, as I wanted to practice with someone who is preparing for the examination at the same time with me.

Dr. O': Where did sit for your examination?

B.J: I sat for the test in Atlanta, Georgia. I think it's much better to sit the examination closer to where you live. I lived in Tampa, Florida at the time. I drove to Atlanta three days ahead of the test, leaving me with adequate time to rest and study.

Dr. O': What about the location for the examination?

B.J: The location was close to my hotel as well, that way I did not have to travel far on the day of the examination. It was a two-minute walk to the test center.

Dr. O': I have heard some people say that some test centers are more favorable than others in terms of passing the examination. What do you think?

B.J: I am not sure that's correct. I have heard people say people fail at the Atlanta Center, but I took my test at the same center and passed the first time.

Dr. O': Could you be an exception, or is it due to your level of preparation?

B.J: I doubt if that is the case. I can share a personal story of a friend who acted based on what she heard on the favorable pass rate at the Philadelphia center. Even though she could have sat for the test in Atlanta since it was close to her, she travelled all the way to the Philadelphia center. When she failed twice at that test center, she decided to give the Atlanta center a try, where she finally passed at the first try.

Dr. O': What is your experience of the examination? Is it a fair test?

B.J: Yes, I think it was fair enough. I had twelve cases in total, consisting six African- Americans and 6 Caucasians. The standardized patients were also well distributed in terms of their age brackets. There was adequate time allotted to introducing the examination prior to its commencement, including an additional five minutes to familiarize yourself with the equipment you will be using for the patients during the examination- like the otoscope, ophthalmoscope, including how to operate the patients' beds.

Dr. O': Did you have any challenges during the examination?

B.J**:** Yes I did. I was very nervous at the start of the examination. I even forgot to summarize and conclude before the bell rang on the first three cases. But I decided I would not to give up and made up my mind that I was going to pass the examination.

Dr. O': How did you do that?

B.J: Right in the middle of the examination, I made a quick readjustment and maintained a heightened focus as I worked through the remaining part of the examination.

Dr. O': What about the issue of time management during the examination?

B.J: Like the other USMLE examinations in general, time is not your friend. That is why endless practice is very important in the few weeks preceding the examination.

Dr. O': What would you tell someone heading to one of the centers next week to take the test?

B.J: It is important to note that one must not leave any stone untouched during the examination. Courtesy and good patient-doctor rapport is vital. Other essential aspects of the examination to pay attention to include good-history taking, focused examination, spending few seconds to give the patient a good summary and conclusion of what you think might be wrong. These aspects form the core of the examination as each one of them forms the basis of your assessment. There is no point concentrating on history taking, while other parts suffer.

Remember courtesy and its value during this component of the examination - don't forget to knock before entering a patient's room in your bid to beat time. Be conscious of time and manage it carefully. Each case will require you to spend fifteen minutes on the history taking, focused examination, summary, and conclusion. Typing the notes will require another ten minutes. Time run so fast!!! This is why one cannot overemphasize the essence of practice.

Dr. O': Is there anything else that you think I am yet to ask?

B.J: One more thing I just remembered, whatever you do not document even though you asked during the patient encounter is judged against you. The same thing applies to elicited tests during the encounter that is not documented.

Dr. O': Any final words on what other people trying to write the CS examination might find useful?

B.J: Hmmm, practice, practice and practice. If you have no practice partner, look for a mannequin. For someone who requires the test scores for an upcoming residency application, remember to schedule your test on time. Available dates are often very limited, especially in the fall. I believe with the right preparation and a good spirit, you can do it.

Dr. O': Thank you B.J, I am sure one, or two people will gain from your experience.

B.J: You are welcome. My pleasure.

Interview #4

This is a transcript of an interview I had with S.D, an international medical graduate who recently passed Step 3 of the United States Medical Licensing Examination (USMLE).

Dr. O': Hello SD, congratulations on successfully completing your steps.

S.D: Thank you sir. Feels so good to be ECFMG certified.

Dr. O': Can you share what helped in your preparation for the Step 3 examination?

S.D: Sure. It was the best idea to write Step 3 when I did, about three months after sitting for the Step 2 CK examination. I did so simply because I didn't want to forget the knowledge I gathered while preparing for the Step 2 CK. So timing is important! Some people will say, since I can always do it during residency, why the rush? But I'm happy I wrote it when I did; that way I do not have to add that to my burden during residency training.

Dr. O': So it is easier to complete the test soon after completing the other steps of the examination.

S.D: It' s definitely easier when you are still in the examination mood.

Dr. O': Can you share the specifics of what you did in your preparation effort?

S.D: These are the steps I took when I was ready to take Step 3?

1. I read the original USMLE Step 3 orientation material on www.usmle.org
2. I registered for the examination online - www.fsmb.org
3. I familiarized myself with the CCS software and the computer-based case simulations.

4. I then put some effort into collating the resources for use in my preparation.

Dr. O': What resources are you talking about?

S.D: I started with USMLE Step 3 practice materials; I mean online sample practice questions. Some of the books I got include Crush Step 3 and Master the Board Step 3. I also subscribed to the U World Step 3 Q bank. Some of my friends used the Archer USMLE online site in their preparation.

Dr. O': So how long did it take you to prepare for the examination?

S.D: Three months.

Dr. O': What kind of questions did you encounter during the examination?

S.D: It was a consecutive two-day examination.

- Day 1 consisted of six blocks of 43 multiple-choice questions to be completed over a period of eight hours, with forty-five minutes break and a fifteen-minute tutorial time. It is possible to skip the tutorial and add that time to the break.
- Day 2 consisted of six blocks of 33 questions each followed by thirteen cases

to be completed over a period of eight hours.

Dr. O': I want you to talk more about the formats of the questions.

S.D: The examination had some drug-ad questions. I would advise that you leave these questions till the end of the block. Some of these questions are time wasting.
There are also statistic questions, some of which may require you to review your Step 1 Statistic review book.

Dr. O': Talk some more about the questions.

S.D: Basically the examination tests ones ability to make the diagnosis, and decide on the management of cases as quickly as possible. The examination was designed to test your ability to perform focused physical assessment especially in emergency situations. You also need to know when to admit a patient to the ICU, or a regular hospital ward.

Dr. O': Considering the challenges relating to time management. How did you go about completing the examination in set time?

S.D: You need to know the relevant and fundamental laboratory tests to order, and which of the tests you can skip to save time and still make your diagnosis, and not delay management. Aim for the minimum practical laboratory tests to make your management decisions. Do not forget basic aspects of care, like remembering to take consent in the course of treating your patient, checking trough level on patients treated with Vancomycin 24 hours after starting treatment, and taking note of the reproductive age of women and completing pregnancy tests on patients who may be exposed to teratogens.

Dr. O': Anything else?

S.D: It's all I can remember.

Dr. O': Thanks for the tips.

S.D: You are welcome.

Becoming Competitive - Am I good enough?

As the number of applicants increases disproportionately to the available positions for residency training, it is imperative that you think ahead of time of a strategy that will allow you to stand out among a pool of applicants. Apart from securing a good score in your performance at the United States Medical Licensing Examination (USMLE), there are many initiatives that you can take well before you start applying for residency positions. A lot of the program directors that run residency programs may not have heard of your medical school of graduation, and you and many others are usually lumped together as graduates of the 'school of international medical graduates'. In other words, your school of graduation is not likely to offer you any major advantage over a fellow international medical graduate.

What you do after you graduate from medical school matters a lot in your preparation for residency training in the United States. While a majority of international medical graduates end up completing an internship, or housemanship following graduation, some end up completing an extra year of national service depending on the country of origin. In those first two years following graduation, a lot depends on where you end up finding yourself. Beyond the first two years, you need to have a plan.

It is important to spend some time to learn about the various medical specialties that are available for training in the United States, and to study what percentage of international medical graduates end up in such specialties. Such information can be readily found in the research section of the United States Medical Licensing Examination (USMLE) website - http://www.usmle.org/data-research/

Additional information can be obtained at the National Resident matching Program website - http://www.nrmp.org/match-data/main-residency-match-data/

These two sites provide you with research materials that reveal current trends and offer you access to historical data that may give you a better understanding of residency training programs and the odds for international medical graduates securing positions in the various medical specialties. The relevance of this information is often missed by many international graduates who have ambitions to pursue a certain specialty, and do so in such a fixated manner without consideration for the limitations posed by the fact that they are graduates of a medical school outside of the territory of the United States and Canada. The majority of international medical graduates end up in residency positions in internal medicine and family practice. This trend is a fairly consistent pattern that hardly changes from year to year. Residency training in surgical specialties are not impossible to secure although as an international medical graduate, you must be willing to alter your plan whenever the odds are no more in your favor. In order not to become distracted from the main theme of this book, I will discuss the subject of training specialty selection in more details in one of the latter chapters of this book.

With respect to what you can do to make yourself attractive as a candidate for residency training, there is no better way to demonstrate this than in this short story that tells of the experience of a husband and wife who arrived in the United States in early 2012. The story of this couple reveals the different paths that the two individuals took in their efforts to improve the chances of securing positions for residency training.

On a dreary Saturday morning in early March 2012, I joined a group of amateur soccer players for a yearly tournament played out between a total of eight teams. I was in no good shape to play competitive soccer with the athletes, many of whom are half my age. I was there in a much safer, but equally important capacity – as a physician with the duty to take care of any one that sustains an injury. I had my First Aid kit with me as usual, and was dressed in a tracksuit ready for the task. Apart from the wet weather, and the accompanying irritating intermittent sprinkles, every other thing seems fine. The soccer matches were played at a local high school athletic field somewhere in Braintree, the same location used in previous years since the tournament began over four years ago. With a total of four groups of two teams, the aim of the tournament was to select the best two teams through a process of elimination that Saturday, and then schedule a final soccer game in the following week.

As I waited for the tournament to begin, I said a silent prayer and hoped that the day will be free of injury. The game started at nine in the morning, with just a few spectators, mostly finally members. It was the usual pattern of spectator attendance, as the majority prefers to wait until the final game a week later to attend. The first set of games was uneventful and four of the teams were already eliminated. Despite the wetness of the grass, there was no single injury. There was a forty-minute break before the next game was scheduled to start, so there was ample time to roam around and interact with the athletes. That was the moment I met Ryan and Betsy – a married couple who had emigrated from Dublin to pursue postgraduate medical training in the United States.

Ryan's team had lost its game and he had nothing else to do but to watch the rest of the tournament. He later told me the bold sign on the First Aid kit bag I was carrying on my shoulder attracted him. He introduced himself and Betsy and told me he had arrived in the December of the year before into the United States. Ryan had a very ebullient personality, and despite the fact that his team had just lost, he seemed very excited for the best team. Betsy was the opposite of Ryan, quiet and reserved. They both offered to join me as I played my part in covering the rest of the tournament for injuries. Throughout the tournament, there was nothing in the way of injuries to manage, so we talked and cheered the players until the best two teams were selected. At the end of the tournament later that day, Ryan offered me an invitation to their apartment for dinner two weeks later, on a Sunday afternoon.

As it was my second time of meeting the two of them, the first being at the soccer tournament two weeks before, I wanted to know more about them and their plans for the future. They were very generous in sharing their plans with me, for reasons that was not quite clear at the time.

Ryan had visited the United States once at the invitation of an uncle six months earlier, and had met a nurse at a local pub at the South End in Boston. It was at that meeting that the thought of coming over to the United States for postgraduate studies occurred to him. He had the luxury of having an uncle who was willing to house him until he settles, so rather than look for any form of employment, he had saved enough money before his arrival and brought enough to cover his expenses in his first few months. The same nurse that he met at the pub also introduced him to a renowned physician - a neurologist, at one of the teaching hospital in Boston, during his first visit. After he returned back to Dublin, he continued to exchange emails with the physician who later offered him an unpaid internship at a research laboratory connected to the hospital.

By the time he finally arrived in Boston, he already had a place to stay, and had an internship position waiting. He also had the fortune of having the offer of the necessary immigration visa by the hospital. Without having any prior experience of basic research in neurology, he put all his energy into learning as much as possible right from the onset. Not only was he able to participate in many of the research studies taking place at the time, he was also able to attend conferences that took place locally, and on one occasion, was selected to make a presentation of one of the research studies he had worked on. At that point in time, he had already made a commitment to follow the path of the physician that invited him over to the United States, and become a neurologist himself. It was at one of those conferences that he met another physician, a program director of an Internal Medicine program, who later offered him an interview for a residency position.

Betsy's experience was the opposite of Ryan. She had come with Ryan, the second time once he made up his mind to come to Boston. Unfortunately for her, she returned back to Dublin after four weeks, as the transition was too much for her to bear. She was an only child, and she felt she had to be with her mother who was suffering from terminal breast cancer, and had not much time to live. She was meant to return to Boston after about a month, but she ended up staying over for six and a half months until her mother succumbed to her illness. During that time, Ryan made two trips to visit Betsy and to see his mother-in-law. Betsy used the time while she was back at home in Dublin to complete some of the United States Medical Licensing Examinations. She later joined Ryan, shortly before he commenced medical residency training.

For the first time, they both left Boston and headed to the Midwest. They were there until Ryan completed his residency training. In the time while Ryan was completing his residency training, Betsy became pregnant and they had their first child - a son. She was at home with her baby until the final year of Ryan's medical residency training when she recruited a babysitter and started applying for residency positions. While she completed the remaining components of the United States Medical Licensing Examinations (USMLE), she was able to secure a position for an internship at the same hospital where Ryan was undergoing his training, but in the psychiatry specialty. Even though she had no interest in psychiatry, it was the only department that would offer her an internship position. Even though she did not like psychiatry as a specialty at first, she gradually developed a liking, and was offered an extension beyond the initial duration of internship by the program director.

Ryan on the other hand, got an offer to complete additional training to complete his certification in neurology at the same hospital where he completed his medical residency. Betsy was concerned about the possibility of separation and had no interest in raising their son far away from his father. She took the unusual step in her effort to secure a residency training position. She went to the psychiatry department were she had recently completed an internship and requested a meeting with the program director. She presented her case with respect to their young child and her concern for family separation knowing that her husband would remain at that same hospital for some more years. The initial response from the program director was that nothing could be done outside of the 'Match', and that there is no guarantee of a position. She did not give up despite the initial rejection. She then went over to meet the program director of the department where her husband was due to commence additional training to become a neurologist. There she presented her case on the grounds of having a young family and her worry over family separation if she had to pursue residency training in another part of the United States. After the meeting, nothing concrete was promised.

After waiting for a period of time without getting any favorable outcome, she gave up on her hope for her desire to materialize. While she was putting all the materials together to apply for residency position elsewhere, she got a call from the psychiatry program director. When she finally met up with her, she was told that for the first time in the history of the program, they have decided to offer her a residency training position outside of the 'Match'. She was so elated that she gave up her dream to be a dermatologist. After the completion of their training, they both decided to return to Boston, where Betsy was likely to have the support of Ryan's uncle and other extended family members in raising their son.

Our meeting ended much later than planned, and ran well into the evening, before we decided to call it a day. I thanked them for sharing their stories with me before I departed.

TIPS/LESSONS

There is no doubt that a little bit of assistance goes a long way in furthering everyone's career ambition. To me, the most important lesson in this story is the power of networking and how much headache you can save yourself by talking to people that you come across in your routine daily encounters. Meeting people is not just enough, letting them know where you need help is more important, as you never know who has the answer until you bring it to their notice.

In the case of Ryan, he was quick to jump at the opportunity presented by a casual contact, and take it further through a consistent communication effort until he was able to get something tangible out of the relationship. A research opportunity is a fantastic opportunity to get into the system, as it provides direct access to a tertiary, or research facility and throws you in the midst of the same group of people that run some of the residency training programs.

In the case of Betsy, she quickly learned how to work the system, by leveraging her husband's relationship to further her agenda. The lesson here is that she is proactive and did not wait for her husband to work on her behalf. She realized the opportunity that she had early and found a way to use it to her advantage. Securing an internship, or an observership position is another alternative way to make useful contacts in addition to acquiring relevant clinical experience. Such experiences not only come in handy during the interview for residency positions, but it is your best chance of securing a supporting reference letter by a clinician based in the United States, an essential requirement of the residency application process.

The remaining section of this chapter is a transcript of a Q & A session of a seminar on the subject of 'Becoming a Desirable Residency Applicant'.

Moderator A.C: Morning to you all. I am glad we all arrived on time. Please be seated. This session is a condensed version of one of our full-day seminars, designed to give you the opportunity to ask questions and have a team of moderators respond to them. This session will be limited to a total of ten questions, after which we will adjourn.

Question #1: It is eight years since I graduated from medical school. I have great scores in the USMLE, but I have not been successful in securing interviews in the last four years. Is it still worthwhile to keep applying?

Panel Member B.D: Even though it is widely talked about, I have not come across any material document that clearly states that an international medical graduate that qualified more than eight years ago is disqualified from participating in the 'Match'. Having said that, it is not impossible for individual programs to have their set policies, both in the written and unwritten form that may pose such limitations. While it is hard to say that you should give up on further attempts to apply to residency training programs, it is not unreasonable to consider alternative career pathways that will enable you to still apply your background in Medicine. While you pursue such alternative career, you can continue in your effort to apply to residency programs in the hope that an opportunity might open up.

Panel Member L.N: With respect to the last question, you have to consider a different approach in your application process, different from the other applicants who are recent medical school graduates. Since you have great scores in the USMLE, I will consider reaching out to residency programs, several months before the normal application process. You may be even make a visit to one, or two programs with a good track record of accepting international medical graduates to see if they would consider you based on your performance and relevant clinical experience. My recommendation is that you do not give up, but to consider a different approach. While you are still in the process, secure a job in medical research as that will keep you closer to the field, and make you an attractive applicant for the right training program.

Question #2: I am visiting the USA briefly and plan to return to Nigeria in two weeks where I am currently in a surgical training program. I plan to apply for residency training I the United States while I am still in training in Nigeria. Am I at a disadvantage?

Panel Member A.C: Nothing is impossible. I have encountered a candidate that did exactly that and successfully matched while still in a training program in another country. I believe with appropriate guidance and counseling it is possible, especially if you score well in the USMLE tests. One caution I will exercise in your case is that you may not necessarily match into a surgical residency program, just because there are relatively fewer positions compared to specialties like Internal Medicine, or Family Practice.

Question #3: What is the ideal length of an internship, or observership to be of significance in your application to a residency program?

Panel Member L.N: There is really no ideal duration for an internship, as it all depends on the nature of the internship, and your level of participation. A lot of internships do not add much to your base knowledge, especially when you are not engaged in the care of a patient. In my experience, I have found the value of an internship to diminish after the fourth week. Before you embark on one, you need to determine what your aims are, and find out what the person in charge is willing to provide. The key is that the right internship will help you with your clinical decision making skills, and offer you a chance to obtain a reference letter from a local physician. Unfortunately, in many instances, it is very difficult for anyone to make a good judgment of you as a person in such a short interval.

Question #4: I plan to apply to General Surgery and Psychiatry at the same time, using two separate personal statements and sets of reference letters. Am I likely to hurt my chances of securing a position?

Panel Member Q.N: In my experience, I have seen that scenario play out in the case of a candidate submitting applications for both Family Practice and Psychiatry. While I understand the need to want to diversify, I also worry that you may lose out on both, as it is often easy to tell where your heart is at the time of your interview. Like the other panel member stated earlier, anything is possible. My advice is that you tread with caution.

Question #5: I have a friend who recently commenced a Masters degree study program. How much weight is put on such endeavors?

Panel Member L.N: There are two instances where this route is considered appropriate. One is when you utilize that route to secure a visa to enter and reside in the United States. The second instance is when it is embarked upon once you have completed the USMLE examinations and while you are waiting to apply for a residency program. There is really no clear data that it offers a clear advantage when you have a great score in the examinations and you have excellent letters of recommendation.

Question #6: Even though the last panel member is not convinced that a Masters degree study program offers any significant advantage, what is the ideal study program to pursue if you have to do so?

Panel Member A.C: My recommendation is that you pursue a subject that interests you as an individual. I have encountered candidates who studied public health, basic sciences, statistics, and even business over the years. I personally have not seen it make much difference when you have a great USMLE test scores and you have strong supporting reference letters. Also remember to consider the cost of such postgraduate education in the long run. Except in a situation where it offers you the advantage to reside temporarily in the United States, I will think twice before incurring such an expense.

Question #7: In addition to having a strong letter of reference from the director of the research laboratory where I currently work, I also had another professor send an email to the program director of a program I am interested in. How often does that work?

Panel Member L.N: In terms of securing an interview, it is definitely likely to help. It all depends on the relationship that exists beforehand. While it may get you through the door for an interview, it may not secure you a position in the program as many factors come into play in the selection of candidates, with more than one person involved in the decision-making.

Question #8: One of my classmates is currently the Chief Resident in a residency program that I am interested in. Is it appropriate to contact her, and if so, how much influence will she have.

Panel Member L.N: Outside of securing you an interview, there is little that she can do. I would definitely reach out to her to see what she can do. Getting an interview allows you that opportunity to prove yourself, and show that you are better than the average candidate.

Question #9: How many applications should I submit to get an interview?

Panel Member A.C: In general, I would say it all depends on your performance in the USMLE. If you have a great score, I would limit it to 25 applications. I once encountered a candidate with mediocre scores that applied to 45 training programs, before getting the one interview that eventually offered her a training position. Remember the cost of submitting the applications, and the cost of travel and hotel accommodation when you have to attend interviews.

Question #10: If you have to advice an applicant about to apply for a residency program one year ahead of time, what would be your recommendation?

Panel Member A.C: If I have the opportunity to work with an applicant one year ahead of time, I will place my effort on ensuring that the candidate work on their USMLE scores and seek opportunities for an internship position that is likely to yield strong letters of reference.

Panel Member L.N: I will have the candidate decide on a few programs that he, or she is interested in, and find a way to contact those programs ahead of time to express an interest, even before submitting a general application.

Panel Member Q.N: For an international medial graduate, I will advice that you select a medical specialty that offers you the best opportunities for interviews and apply to as many programs as you can afford.

Panel Member B.D: I will pay a lot of attention to the personal statement and the letters of recommendation. I will try to research IMG-friendly residency programs and apply to those programs first, before applying to others.

Moderator A.C: This session could easily run for another two hours. To the members of the panel, I thank you for your contribution. To the attendees, I thank you for being a great audience. I wish you the best of luck as you apply for residency positions.